REVERSE TYPE 2 DIABETES MADE EASY

How To Reverse Type 2 Diabetes In 30 Days By Losing Weight And Eating The Right Food

Happy Health Publishing

THANK YOU FOR YOUR PURCHASE!

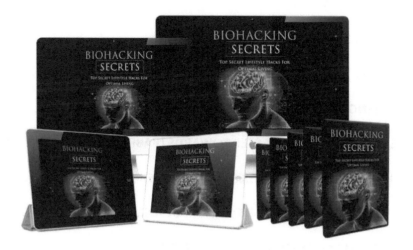

DO YOU LIKE HAPPY HEALTH PUBLISHING?
SUBSCRIBE TO OUR NEWSLETTER AND
DOWNLOAD YOUR FREE GIFT NOW!

IT WILL HELP YOU LIVE YOUR BEST LIFE AND

CLAIM YOUR PERSONAL POWERS!

https:// l.ead.me/hhp-free-gift

TABLE OF CONTENTS

LIST OF FIGURES

INTRODUCTION

Diabetes is a leading health concern throughout the world. Millions of people live with diabetes and the tally goes up with the additions of millions more every year. According to the International Diabetes Federation's report of 2019, the total number of diabetic patients around the world is estimated to be 463 million and by the looks of statistics and graphs, this number is expected to increase up to 700 million by the end of 2045. While type 1 Diabetes is also significant, diabetes type 2 makes up more than 90% of the total diabetic cases globally.

LIFESTYLE AND OBESITY

Lifestyle and obesity have a significant co-relation with Type 2 diabetes. A sedentary lifestyle with restricted physical activity is a leading cause of many pathologies including cardiovascular diseases and diabetes. Over the last couple of decades, obesity has also evolved as a global health concern because it is a serious risk factor for diabetes(1). The frequency of obesity has nearly doubled during the last decade. According to a report that evaluated the prevalence of obesity among people in 2014, nearly 39 percent of people who were 18 years or older were overweight and 13 percent were obese (1). Obesity is evaluated on WHO BMI charts with values of 30-35,35-40 and above 40 of great concern (morbidly obese). Most cases of obesity are associated with **high caloric intake, high fat consumption, limited or no physical activity,** and a sedentary work routine(2). Because of its direct association with the development of insulin resistance in the body, obesity is a common underlying cause of T2DM (Type 2 Diabetes Mellitus). According to WHO, obesity accounts for 44% of the diabetic cases, and obesity-associated diabetic cases are expected to rise to 300 million by end of 2025. The close association between obesity and T2DM has allowed physicians to explore the non-pharmacological management of diabetes by adjusting and modulating the diet and physical activity factor for disease control(1).

BREAKING THE PROGRESSIVE CYCLE

The symptoms of diabetes include polyuria (frequent urination), polydipsia (increased thirst), and polyphagia (increased hunger) because the cells are unable to use glucose as an energy source and are starved(3). Other symptoms include blurred vision, fatigue, and a hyperglycemic state associated with a decreased level of consciousness. It's important to break the progressive cycle for effective management of the disease. The cycle starts with high blood glucose levels (such as after a meal) to which the insulin response is inadequate. Because insulin resistance is a dominant feature in type 2 diabetes, more insulin is released from the pancreas to compensate for tissue's insensitivity to insulin. This raises insulin levels in the blood and because one of the effects of insulin is to promote fat synthesis (lipogenesis), increased fat deposition causes weight gain and obesity that leads to further insulin resistance in the body. The increased workload on the pancreas to secrete excess insulin causes damage to pancreatic cells which then creates insulin deficiency and high blood glucose levels responsible for the symptoms of diabetes.

Fortunately, it is possible to reverse this cycle by adjusting diet and lifestyle besides pharmacological management of type 2 diabetes. Because high caloric intake combined with restricted or no physical activity is the root cause of obesity-associated diabetes, replacing high-calorie fatty meals with a low-calorie yet healthy diet and at the same time ensuring regular exercise and a physically active work routine can be used for effective management of type 2 diabetes(4).

WEIGHT LOSS; THE FIRST STEP TOWARDS DIABETIC REVERSAL

Weight loss is a solution to a lot of health problems including cardiovascular diseases and diabetes. Especially for type 2 diabetic patients, weight loss is extremely crucial for disease remission and reversal. Losing several pounds can significantly impact disease management and prognosis but putting off weight isn't that easy. So, how can weight loss be achieved efficiently without having to engage in strenuous exercises? The answer lies in adjusting diet and doing little but consistent physical activity and exercise (at least a few minutes every day)(4). This will prevent weight regain once you have managed to lose weight. Most weight loss aspirants have a yearning to lose all their extra fat in one day. They go for rigorous exercise rather than tweaking their diet and supplementing it with light exercise. So, it's important to acknowledge that weight loss is a **steady process that requires consistent effort.** It's best to start with small steps instead of steaming up things in a single day. A regular walk around the block every day is a good start for weight loss. Once it becomes easy to achieve these small milestones every day, things can be stepped up such as replacing the walk with brisk walking and then with jogging or perhaps increasing the mileage. Being active and increasing the span of **everyday physical activity is key to losing weight** and healthier life. According to the [National Weight Control registry](), 90% of the people who achieved their weight loss goals reported at least half an hour of exercise every day (with walking being the exercise for most of these people).

Diet: Besides exercise, the other important factor for weight loss is diet. Diet should be adjusted and scheduled. It's advisable no to skip breakfasts because this leads to overeating later in the day that significantly dampens your weight loss efforts. Breakfast should be done regularly and include healthy carbohydrates (those with low glycemic index), fibers, eggs, and whole grains. Foods with added sugars should be avoided. It is very important to restrict the total caloric intake for weight loss. Calories can be reduced by **replacing starchy vegetables** with green vegetables and proteins (in type 2 diabetic patients). High use of fibers is recommended because of their high satiety value. Fibers slow the digestion process and help control blood glucose levels. They are highly recommended for cutting calories. A study from The Journal of Nutrition (published in 2019) showed that individuals who consumed fibers were better able to cut calories and lose weight.

OTHER VALUABLE STRATEGIES TO LIMIT OVER-EATING

It is important to limit overeating and prevent untimed cravings for food. To prevent eating a lot, it is recommended to start a meal with non-starchy vegetables(5). They are low in calories and do not affect your blood glucose levels significantly and by the time you get to other foods, you already have a feeling of being full. Another useful trick to avoid over-eating is to prepare a kind of broth of your salad dressings and dipping the salad into it instead of sprinkling the dressing on the salad. Though it seems unrealistic, this technique induces early satiety and helps restrict the total caloric consumption. It's also advisable to keep oneself busy in some activity because being idle increases the chances of eating without having the real urge to eat.

Once you have lost weight, it's essential to maintain it by following a strict schedule. Maintaining a diet and exercising regularly keeps the weight off and is really crucial to people living with type w diabetes.

FOODS THAT HELP REVERSE TYPE 2 DIABETES

Having a correct diet can help reverse type w diabetes and avoid its complications. A perfect diet for this purpose includes carbohydrates, fats, and proteins all in the correct ratio. Carbohydrates targeted for reversing diabetes are those of a low glycemic index (that defines how quickly a carbohydrate can raise your blood glucose levels)(5). Similarly, plant-derived fats are recommended in the nutrition architecture for diabetic reversal. Carbohydrates usually recommended for diabetic patients are complex carbohydrates (with low glycemic index and load). These carbohydrates are taken as a part of whole food mixed with other components like fibers, vitamins, and proteins that not only slow down the absorption of such carbohydrates but also prevent rapid rises in blood glucose levels and thus aid in glycemic control. Some common complex carbohydrates recommend as a diet for type 2 diabetic patients are

1. whole wheat
2. brown rice

3. quinoa

4. Fruits and vegetables

5. Beans

6. lentils.

PROTEINS RECIPES FOR DIABETIC REVERSAL

Proteins also are an important source of energy. The overall absorption and release of energy from proteins is a little slower process but the fact that proteins do not alter the blood glucose levels makes them a good choice for diabetic patients. Proteins also have a high satiety value and help deal with hunger and random cravings. Plant proteins are generally preferred over animal proteins. Protein intake can be ensured through **various savory recipes** described below

Eggs: Eggs are perhaps the most widely consumed products globally because of the wide range of recipes and different styles that they offer to their consumers. You can have **an omelet, fried egg, boiled egg**; even a mashed egg would serve the purpose. Eggs are a rich source of protein and highly efficient food choices for diabetic patients(5). They should be taken with every meal because they'll help with keeping the blood glucose stable and induce satiety. Now when there are different styles you can cook an egg in, a spinach omelet would best serve the purpose of diabetic reversal. This blend of green vegetables and rich proteins (both recommended food choices for reversal of diabetes) would ensure both flavor (for those who like **mouthwatering recipes) and health. To top it off, a spinach omelet sizzling in olive oil** would be so satisfying yet healthy.

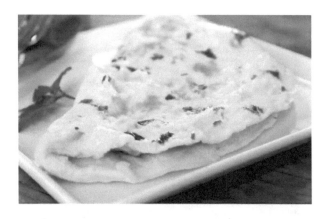

Figure 1: Eggs

Fish: Fish is also a rich source of protein and provides omega-3 fats too(6). While proteins take care of the body's energy requirements and glycemic control, omega-3 fats increase neuronal transmission and sharpness improving overall cognition and memory. You can have fish in abundance without compromising your blood glucose levels.

Fish can be prepared according to taste (can be fried in olive oil, baked, or grilled), and to make it savory without putting any strain on its nutritional benefit for diabetic patients, it can also be seasoned with mixed herbs. Other seafood has equal nutritional benefits and is recommended for use by diabetic patients to help them reverse the condition.

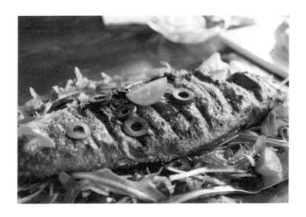

Figure 2: Fish

Have Baked Turkey more often than just thanksgiving.

Other sources of protein ensuring both taste and health benefits are chicken and turkey(6). Chicken can also be prepared in different styles, can be mixed with vegetables, or consumed alone (grilled chicken). One flavorful chicken recipe for diabetic patients could be a grilled chicken sandwich with tender and juicy chicken pressed between whole grain toasts and seasoned with some herbs and lettuce. Chicken provides proteins containing all the essential amino acids required by the body and also aids in managing blood glucose levels. It also has a high satiety value. Turkey on the other hand also provides the body with **proteins enriched with all the essential amino acids.** A tantalizing Turkey recipe for diabetic patients (without compromising glucose levels) could be a **turkey baked with light spices and soy sauce.** The protein content will keep the blood glucose level stable while the recipe would provide a satisfying taste without compromising health benefits.

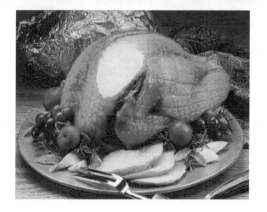

Figure 3: Turkey

Other protein diets recommended for the reversal of type 2 diabetes should include sources such as **beans, legumes, peas, tofu, and soy foods**. It's important to plan a meal by paying attention to the proportions of fats, proteins, and carbohydrate content. Because fats, proteins, and fibers increase the absorption time of carbohydrates and lower the glycemic index of a carb diet, it's important to have them in adequate content in the meal to ensure this glycemic control benefit for diabetic patients.

CARBOHYDRATE CONSUMPTION FOR DIABETIC PATIENTS

Green Vegetable Recipes are a Good Choice. Green vegetables are a really good choice for diabetic patients. These vegetables can be consumed in excess without having to worry about their glycemic effects on the body(7). These vegetables are generally non-starchy and do not have a significant effect on resting blood glucose levels (due to low glycemic index). They contain all the essential vitamins and other nutrients to refuel your body. These green vegetables are preferred over starchy vegetables such as potatoes that have a high glycemic index and are only recommended in restricted quantities to diabetic patients. Green vegetables have the added benefit of reducing body fat and obesity and taking down another important morbidity that comes with diabetes. To add a **bit of flavor to these vegetables** and to avoid a monotonous diet, green vegetables can be **seasoned with herbs** (both fresh and dried), **vinaigrette dressing, or olive oil**. Try consuming a lot of green vegetables if you have diabetes and see the change.

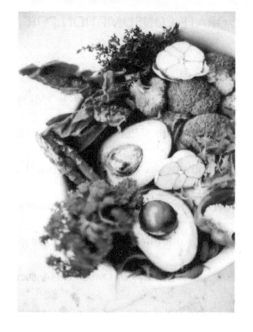

Figure 4: Green Vegetables

CONSUME WHOLE GRAINS

Grains are always preferred for diabetic patients because of twofold benefits: they have a low glycemic index and do not impact blood glucose levels much. 2- When consumed with a high-carb diet, grains such as **brown rice or quinoa** decrease the absorption of carbohydrates and contribute to lowering your blood glucose levels(8). It is important to consume whole grains regularly and to make sure if you taking them in the form of whole-grain bread, that each slice contains **greater than three grams** of whole grain.

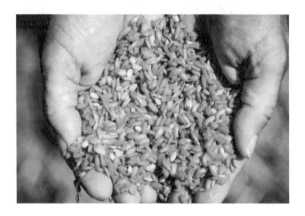

Figure 5: Whole Grains

FATS THAT SHOULD BE CONSUMED IF YOU HAVE DIABETES

Fats are high reservoirs of energy. One gram of fats provides the body with nearly 9kcal of energy (the kind of energy required by the starving cells). Fats do not affect your blood glucose levels but they do contribute to glycemic control by slowing down the absorption of carbohydrates when taken with them as a meal. But not all fats are good. Fats of animal origin pose a threat to the body by increasing the risk for cardiovascular diseases. However, **dairy fats like yogurt are extremely helpful for diabetic patients.** Major oils that should be taken for reversing type 2 diabetes are plant oils like:

1. Olive oil

2. Nut oil

3. Avocado

These are not associated with risk for cardiovascular diseases. Instead, they increase circulating HDL (high-density lipoprotein) levels that are good for health. Fish oil is another thing that is recommended for diabetic reversal with the added benefit of improving synaptic transmission and cognition (because fish contains omega-3 fats that enhance neuronal transmission). Healthy fats also have a high satiety value that can help decrease hunger and reduce cravings for carbohydrates(6). **All you need is to sit back and enjoy an avocado-soaked whole-grain toast (both healthy and satisfying to your taste buds) as a part of your diet therapy for diabetic reversal.**

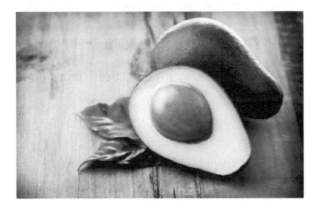

Figure 6: Avocado

MEAL PLANS FOR TYPE 2 DIABETIC PATIENTS

Meal plans for diabetic reversal vary from person to person. However, a general rule is to pay special focus to the content of different nutritional ingredients. An ideal meal should include a lot of vegetables (especially green and non-starchy) and a limited number of sugars and red meat. A reduced amount of carbohydrate content in the meal is essential to prevent any rapid rise in blood glucose levels.

VEGAN DIET

For people with type 2 diabetes, a vegetarian diet is an excellent option for disease reversal(7) and remission. The diet includes lots of green vegetables supplemented with proteins and plant oils. This diet should ideally include 1- fruits and vegetables 2-high quality proteins from beans, legumes, peas, nuts, and seeds 3- high-quality plant fats such as olive oil and avocado 4-whole grains such as brown rice rather than processed starches sugars.

This kind of vegan diet is rich in essential nutrients and fibers has low caloric value, and is also lower in saturated fats. The effectiveness of such a diet for type 2 diabetic patients is supported by research studies.

ADA DIET FOR DIABETES

American diabetic association describes the macronutrient ratio for a diabetic diet. According to it, the meal should include complex carbohydrates that can be obtained from brown rice and it should be supplemented with whole grains and protein. The fat content of the meal should be from unsaturated fats. Sugars and sweetened beverages should be avoided in particular. The ADA also recommends physical activity and exercise along with diet for effective diabetic reversal.

PALEO DIET

Paleolithic diet refers to a primitive diet pattern much like the diet of the people who lived in the stone age. It focuses on the protein content along with fruits, vegetables, and other natural sources. According to studies, one major reason for growing diseases in our generation is an imbalanced diet. Our systems have not evolved to accommodate calorie-dense meals that we eat followed by limited or no physical activity. The sedentary lifestyle and a high-caloric intake lead to more fate synthesis and storage in our body causing obesity and its associated health risks. The paleolithic diet recommended for diabetic patients includes lean meat, nuts, fruits, vegetables, and unsaturated fats. It avoids sugars, refined fats, soft drinks, grains, and dairy products. This kind of diet has been proved beneficial for diabetic patients by some clinical studies.

MEDITERRANEAN DIET

This type of diet is followed in Italy and Greece (but does not include the Italian pasta of course). Mediterranean diet specializes in **lots of vegetables.** Other components ate **fruits, plant oils, avocado, nuts, and fish.** It may include a small amount of meat and dairy products. The key importance of the diet lies in its nutritional value(9). This type of meal is highly dense in all the essential nutrients required by the body. It not only maintains the blood glucose levels but also helps in weight loss. Both of these aspects are crucial to the reversal of diabetes. There are generally two variants of the Mediterranean diet, depending on the content of olive oil and nuts. However, an ideal diet should include an abundance of both of these ingredients as they play an important role in glycemic control and diabetic remission. To make your meal scrumptious, you can sprinkle chopped almonds on green beans or drizzle zucchini with olive oil, oregano, and hemp seeds. This diet has gained increasing popularity because of its variant flavor and health benefits(9).

IF YOU HAVE TYPE 2 DIABETES, YOU MIGHT WANT TO TRY THESE SUPER FOODS

Superfoods are not only nutritionally rich giving the body all the essential proteins, fats, vitamins, and carbs but these foods also have added health benefits improving the overall functioning of the body(10). Type 2 diabetic patients can benefit from the superfoods described below.

1. **Chia Seeds:** These seeds are rich sources of omega-3 fats, proteins, and soluble fibers. The omega-3 fats in chia seeds improve brain functioning. On the whole, these seeds help stabilize blood glucose levels (by reducing the glycemic load of meals) and induce satiety. These seeds can be consumed in the morning with breakfast to increase their satiety value. The soluble fiber in chia seeds makes them a good thickener to be used in cooking and especially baking. These seeds also have the royalty to be molded into a yummy pudding by mixing them with some cocoa and almond milk. Thus, because of

their healthy ingredients, Chia seeds make a good choice of food for people with type 2 diabetes.

2. **Salmon (wild):** As discussed previously, fish is the best source of protein for diabetic patients in addition to chicken and turkey. Wild salmon because of its high protein content has no effect on raising the blood glucose levels (effective glycemic control). It induces satiety and decreases irregular cravings. Not only this, the high ratio of omega-3 fats to saturated fats in salmon improves neuronal processes and brain functioning (omega-3 fats are good fats with health benefits)(6). It's important to use wild salmon rather than farm salmon because farm fish are higher in organic pollutants and inflammation-inducing chemicals and can be health risks instead of benefiting one's health. So, if you are a type 2 diabetic and are tired of eating vegetables and whole grains, a wild salmon with light spices might no be a bad choice.

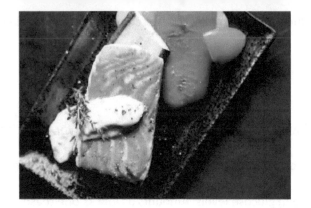

Figure 7: Salmon

3. **White vinegar:** Vinnegar goes without saying to be one of the best ingredients when it comes to enhancing the flavor and aroma of meals. **You can mix your salads with a little vinegar and can use it as an enhancer for your vegetables and chicken recipes.** Vinegar has a special effect of delaying gastric emptying which is highly essential in keeping the blood glucose levels in a steady state. By preventing rapid rises in blood glucose, the insulin response of the body is kept within the normal range and no excess load is out on the pancreas. Vinegar like other superfoods has a high satiety value too. This prevents overeating and significant fluctuations in blood

glucose which makes vinegar consumption an excellent choice for type 2 diabetic patients(10).

4. **Cinnamon:** Cinnamon is also a superfood for diabetic patients because it lowers both fasting and post-prandial (right after a meal) glucose levels. Amounts as low as one teaspoon per day can produce significant health benefits(5). Cinnamon too can be incorporated into a meal in a lot of different ways. It can be sprinkled over preparations to add flavor and color. Adding cinnamon to milk also provides pain relief. The high polyphenol content of cinnamon also avoids any health risks and complications. **Maybe a cinnamon coffee is all you need for your diabetes.**

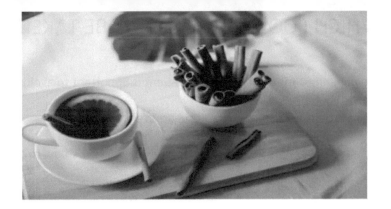

Figure 8: Cinnamon

5. **Lentils:** Another super food with exceptional health benefits is lentils. Lentils contain high quantities of vitamins including the B vitamins such as folic acid. Moreover, lentils are rich in minerals and a perfect ratio of proteins and complex carbohydrates makes them the perfect choice for people with type 2 diabetes. You can lentils cooked or use them in salads. You can also enjoy them in soups (the softer orange and yellow ones). Because lentils also help maintain blood glucose levels, it's advisable to use them frequently as a part of your meal(5).

WHICH FOODS SHOULD NOT BE TAKEN?

While planning a meal for a diabetic patient is important to avoid foods that quickly raise your blood sugar levels. All kinds of sweetened beverages should be completely avoided. It's best to avoid the following things:

- Refined sugars such as sweets and candies
- Dairy products having a high-fat content such as whole milk, cheese, etc.
- Processed carbohydrates such as pasta
- Red meat
- Foods with trans fats such as mayonnaise and other similar spreads

If you are a type 2 diabetic, you should be highly critical of your food choices. Limiting high carbs and shifting towards green vegetables and healthy proteins should be the utmost priority. You should also pay attention to the ingredients of the meal in a restaurant setting while making an order. It's best to ask about the ingredients before making an order. Foods with high content of vegetables and proteins should be given priority on the order list. **Desserts should specifically be avoided while dining out.**

Another important thing to consider is if you can have alcohol. Moderate alcohol consumption reduces the risk for cardiovascular diseases. However, alcohol has the effect of reducing blood sugar levels (causing hypoglycemia) so too much alcohol should be avoided. Alcohol consumption should be kept in check if you are using insulin because alcohol can cause significantly delayed hypoglycemia. The risk for alcohol-induced hypoglycemia can be reduced by taking alcohol with foods.

UNDERSTANDING TYPE 2 DIABETES

Type 2 diabetes is a heterogeneous disease with multiple underlying causes and genetic modulations. Unlike type 1 diabetes mellitus, it does not involve the destruction of pancreatic beta cells. Instead, type 2 diabetes is characterized by an increased insulin resistance by the tissues and subsequent high blood glucose levels. The relative insulin deficiency created because of the inability of the tissues to utilize the hormone accounts for the hyperglycemia type 2 diabetes(3).

INSULIN AND DIABETES

Insulin is a hormone released by beta cells in the pancreas in response to hyperglycemia. High blood glucose levels are sensed by pancreatic glucokinase and glucose enters the beta cells via GLUT-2 (transporters in beta cells membranes). It moves down the glycolytic pathway to yield ATP that causes closure of ATP-sensitive K+ channels and membrane depolarization. This allows the opening up of calcium channels and the release of insulin through exocytosis. Adequate insulin response to hyperglycemia is essential to bring down the glucose levels within the physiological range. Failure to decrease blood glucose levels can create micro and macro-vascular complications. People with type 2 diabetes develop insulin resistance which means their bodies are not able to utilize insulin efficiently. This leads to a build-up of glucose in their bloodstream (3).

GENETIC PREDISPOSITION FOR TYPE 2 DIABETES

Genetic variations and mutations also play a role in the development of the disease(2). More than 250 gene loci have been recognized to play a role in a predisposition towards the disease. Genomic variations result in a complex of beta-cell failure, insulin insensitivity, and loss of the body's glycemic control mechanisms. The genomic architecture of type 2 diabetes involves multiple variations in a number of different genes that contribute to overall disease development and progression. A variant of type 2 diabetes called **maturity-onset diabetes of the young (MODY)** is known to result from mutations in hepatocyte nuclear factor 1 (HNF-1) and glucokinase (GCK) gene(2). The mutations in the glucokinase gene are responsible for defective endogenous insulin secretion and a crippled glycemic control system in such patients. However, T2DM mostly results from polygenetic mutations and variations rather than defects in a single gene. These variations may be epigenetic or may also run in families increasing the risk for disease development dramatically if it is also present in the individual's parents. Linkage studies (studies involving a pattern of inheritance of linked base pairs across the genome from one generation to the other) have identified certain inherited genetic markers linked with disease development. Among these, CAPN10 (involved in receptor modulation and intracellular signaling) and TF7L2 (Transcription factor 7 like 2) are usually associated with type 2 diabetes(2).

COMPLICATIONS OF DIABETES

Type 2 diabetes has a lot of complications **both short-term and long term.** The most common short-term complication of diabetes is hypoglycemia (low blood glucose levels) if a diabetic complication is on insulin(3). The drop in blood sugar levels results because of insulin-induced uptake of glucose by cell. Hypoglycemia after an insulin shot can manifest in the form of rapid heartbeats, sweating, headache, and confusion. It is advisable to some sweet juice or candy after insulin shot to avoid rapid drops in blood glucose levels.

Another short-term complication of diabetes is a **hyperosmolar hyperglycemic state.** The high blood glucose levels (hyperglycemia) as a result of insulin resistance trigger the body's compensatory responses. The most common response is to excrete glucose in urine. Because glucose is an osmotically active substance, it takes a lot of water with it resulting in excessive urination (polyuria). The loss of water further raises blood glucose concentration (hyperosmolar hyperglycemia). This condition can be so severe that it can result in a coma. To avoid this complication, it's important to keep the body

hydrated and monitor blood sugar levels for any spikes.

LONG-TERM COMPLICATIONS OF DIABETES

Long-term complications of diabetes usually arise if it is left untreated and these complications stem from the effect of high sugar levels on blood vessels. Hyperglycemia can target both micro and macro (large) vessels(11). Major small vessels affected by high blood sugar levels are those in the eye. A condition called **diabetic retinopathy** severely affects the visual field and impairs vision. High blood sugar levels can also cause **cataract formation in the eyes**. Other vessels affected by diabetes are those of the kidney that impairs renal function (filtration of blood). You can detect **diabetic kidney** damage in the early stages by monitoring the amount of albumin in the urine. Increased albumin would suggest diabetic nephropathy.

Nerves also suffer a significant amount of damage from persistent hyperglycemia. **Diabetic foot** is a very common condition that stems from peripheral neuropathies caused by diabetes (in the foot). The patient develops sores on the foot without feeling them (due to nerve damage). These sores then grow in size and get infected to an extent that the foot has to be amputated to prevent further infection.

MACROVASCULAR COMPLICATIONS

Type 2 diabetes also affects large blood vessels such s those of the heart and brain. These two organs are the most important organs of the body and any damage to them is potentially fatal. Diabetes leads to plaque formation in these large vessels. In the heart, this is followed by a **heart attack**(11) whereas, in the brain, a stroke pursues. Both of these conditions are life-threatening so it's important to monitor and keep your blood sugar levels in check if you are a type 2 diabetic patient.

ADJUSTING LIFESTYLE AND DIET

Although type 2 diabetes is a rising health concern globally and is accompanied by a lot of life-threatening complications, with a little and consistent effort it can be managed and reversed. Adjusting lifestyle from a sedentary routine to a physically more active schedule can do wonders for diabetic patients. A minimum exercise routine of at least 30 mins per day comprising just light exercise or even simple walking is highly recommended to all people, not just those who suffer from type 2 diabetes. Exercise not only reduces the risk for diabetes and helps people living with the disease but also keeps a lot other cardiovascular diseases away. The second most important thing is to select a healthy diet. Unfortunately, people prefer processed and frozen foods over fresh fruits and vegetables and this is perhaps one of the main reasons for the decreased immune status of the body that renders it vulnerable to a wide spectrum of diseases and complications. One should always have a preference for fresh and healthy food including green vegetables, fresh fruits, whole grains, high-quality fats, and proteins. Meals should be rich in fibers because they not only have a high satiety value but also slow down the absorption process that helps prevent over-eating and rapid rises in blood sugar levels of people with type 2 diabetes. Thus, by simply tweaking your lifestyle and diet, you can significantly improve the quality of your life and reverse your diabetic status. And now that you know the essentials to make possible a diabetic reversal within just 30 days by adjusting your routine and diet, **WASTE NO TIME AND GET TO WORK NOW!**

REFERENCES:

1. Maggio CA, Pi-Sunyer FX. Obesity and type 2 diabetes. Endocrinol Metab Clin North Am. 2003 Dec;32(4):805–22, viii.
2. Fletcher B, Gulanick M, Lamendola C. Risk factors for type 2 diabetes mellitus. J Cardiovasc Nurs. 2002 Jan;16(2):17–23.
3. Taylor R. Type 2 diabetes: etiology and reversibility. Diabetes Care. 2013 Apr;36(4):1047–55.
4. Colberg SR, Sigal RJ, Fernhall B, Regensteiner JG, Blissmer BJ, Rubin RR, et al. Exercise and type 2 diabetes: the American College of Sports Medicine and the American Diabetes Association: a joint position statement. Diabetes Care. 2010 Dec;33(12):e147-67.
5. Forouhi NG, Misra A, Mohan V, Taylor R, Yancy W. Dietary and nutritional approaches for prevention and management of type 2 diabetes. BMJ. 2018 Jun;361:k2234.
6. Westman EC, Tondt J, Maguire E, Yancy WSJ. Implementing a low-carbohydrate, ketogenic diet to manage type 2 diabetes mellitus. Expert Rev Endocrinol Metab. 2018 Sep;13(5):263–72.
7. Barnard ND, Katcher HI, Jenkins DJA, Cohen J, Turner-McGrievy G. Vegetarian and vegan diets in type 2 diabetes management. Nutr Rev. 2009 May;67(5):255–63.
8. Lee Y-M, Kim S-A, Lee I-K, Kim J-G, Park K-G, Jeong J-Y, et al. Effect of a Brown Rice Based Vegan Diet and Conventional Diabetic Diet on Glycemic Control of Patients with Type 2 Diabetes: A 12-Week Randomized Clinical Trial. PLoS One. 2016;11(6):e0155918.
9. Esposito K, Maiorino MI, Bellastella G, Chiodini P, Panagiotakos D, Giugliano D. A journey into a Mediterranean diet and type 2 diabetes: a systematic review with meta-analyses. BMJ Open. 2015 Aug;5(8):e008222.
10. van den Driessche JJ, Plat J, Mensink RP. Effects of superfoods on risk factors of metabolic syndrome: a systematic review of human intervention trials. Food Funct. 2018 Apr;9(4):1944–66.
11. Kehler DS, Stammers AN, Susser SE, Hamm NC, Kimber DE, Hlynsky MW, et al. Cardiovascular complications of type 2

diabetes in youth. Biochem Cell Biol. 2015 Oct;93(5):496–510.

THANK YOU
FOR FINISHING THE BOOK!

We would like to thank you very much for supporting us and reading through to the end. We know you could have picked any number of books to read, but you picked this book and for that, we are extremely grateful.

We hope you enjoyed your reading experience. If so, it would be really nice if you could share this book with your friends and family by posting on Facebook and Twitter.

Happy Health Publishing stands for the highest reading quality and we will always endeavor to provide you with high-quality books.

Would you mind leaving us a review on Amazon before you go?
Because it will mean a lot to us and support us in creating high-quality guidelines for you in the future.

Please help us reach more readers by taking 30 seconds to write just a few words on Amazon now.

Warmly yours,
The Happy Health Publishing Team

IF YOU'VE ENJOYED
REVERSE TYPE 2 DIABETES MADE EASY,
YOU'LL ALSO ENJOY IN THIS SERIES:

EPSTEIN-BARR VIRUS FOR BEGINNERS:

Find out how to Fight The Epstein-Barr Virus And Chronic Fatigue
Syndrome With The Right Treatment Of EBV.

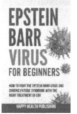 

https://amzn.to/3uuuPQ3*

FUN AND WEIRD MEDICAL FACTS:

10 Amazing Facts About the Human Body You Have Never Thought of.

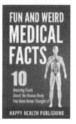 

https://amzn.to/3utQ44u*

THE ANTI-INFLAMMATORY VITAMIN MADE EASY:

A Beginner's Guide On How To Stop Chronic Inflammation With Vitamin D Supplements.

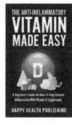 

https://amzn.to/3tE2ZA3*

Made in United States
Troutdale, OR
04/27/2024

19491592R00037